Botanical Beauty

Harnessing the Power of Plants for Healthy Hair

Harmony Royce

DEDICATION

This book is dedicated to everyone who thinks self-care and confidence can change the world.

To those who accept their own beauty and understand that taking care of their hair is a statement of self-love rather than merely a routine.

To the friends, parents, and mentors that encourage us to take care of our bodies and brains and serve as a constant reminder that the path to accepting oneself starts inside.

To all the enthusiastic hair care experts and enthusiasts who never stop learning and imparting their knowledge, enhancing our comprehension of wellness and beauty.

I hope that this book will help everyone on their path to healthier, more gorgeous hair by providing them with motivation, empowerment, and useful advice.

DISCLAIMER

This book's content is not meant to be used as medical advice; rather, it is meant purely for educational and informative reasons. The author and publisher have taken every precaution to ensure the quality and dependability of the material provided; nonetheless, they make no guarantees or claims regarding the content's suitability or completeness.

Before making any big changes to their food, lifestyle, or hair care regimen, readers are advised to speak with licensed healthcare professionals. This is especially important if they already have health conditions or concerns. The author disclaims all obligations for any unfavorable effects or repercussions arising from the use or implementation of the material included herein. Individual results may vary depending on specific circumstances.

There may be references in this book to goods or services that the author, publisher, or other parties do not support or are associated with. When choosing hair care products or treatments, always do extensive research and take individual preferences and sensitivities into consideration.

You recognize and agree to these terms and conditions by reading this book.

CONTENTS

ACKNOWLEDGMENTS

I want to express my sincere appreciation to everyone who helped make this book possible.

I would like to express my gratitude to my family and friends for their constant support and encouragement along this journey. Your support of my vision has always given me motivation.

I am incredibly grateful to the hair care specialists and experts whose wisdom and ideas helped to develop the contents of this book. I'm motivated to spread this knowledge to others by your devotion to teaching and your passion for the art.

A particular thanks goes out to the innumerable people who have offered their personal hair care experiences and stories, which have greatly enhanced the story and added important viewpoints.

I also want to thank all of the sources and in-depth research that helped me write this book. The knowledge presented in these pages has a strong foundation thanks to the efforts of writers, scientists, and hair care professionals.

Finally, I would like to express my gratitude to each and every reader for their interest and time spent learning about hair care. With this book, I wish to empower you on your path to gorgeous, healthy hair.

CHAPTER 1

COMPREHENDING YOUR HAIR

Hair is a sign of one's physical and mental well-being, not only an aesthetic characteristic. Maintaining gorgeous and healthy hair requires an understanding of the structure of the scalp, typical issues that arise, and the significance of scalp health. This chapter delves into the basic components of hair care, covering topics such as the science of hair structure, typical problems, and scalp health.

1.1 THE HUMAN HAIR STRUCTURE

The Function of Hair Follicles in Hair Growth

The microscopic, tunnel-like structures called hair follicles are anchored to the scalp by hair and are found in the dermis, the second layer of skin. The several components that make up each follicle are essential to the development, expansion, and final shedding of hair. These components include:

- **Hair bulb:** The hair shaft is formed by the division and growth of live cells found in the hair bulb, which is situated at the base of the follicle.

- **Dermal papilla:** A ring of blood vessels that lies beneath the hair bulb and supplies oxygen and nutrients to promote the development of hair.

- **Sebaceous gland:** Secretes sebum, a naturally occurring oil that lubricates the scalp and hair to avoid dryness.

There are three stages in the cycle of hair growth:

1. **Anagen:** The first two to six years of growth.

2. **Catagen:** The two to three week transitional period during which hair growth slows.

3. **Telogen:** The period of rest, which lasts for two to four months, during which time hair falls out and new growth

starts.

The Cuticle, Cortex, and Medulla are the Three Layers of Hair

Three separate layers make up hair, and they all affect the structure, strength, and look of the hair:

- **Cuticle:** The outermost layer, made up of cells that overlap and serve as scales for protection. A cuticle in good health is flat and reflects light to provide the appearance of shine. Dullness and tangling are the results of damage to this layer.

- **Cortex:** The cortex, which comprises the majority of the hair shaft, is located beneath the cuticle. Melanin, which gives hair its color, and keratin, a structural protein, are found in the cortex. The strength, flexibility, and texture of the hair are determined by this layer.

- **Medulla:** The deepest layer, present in hair strands with greater thickness. It may contribute to the resilience and insulation of the hair, while its exact role is unknown.

The Distinction Between Damaged and Healthy Hair

Adequate hydration, a robust internal structure, and a smooth cuticle are the hallmarks of healthy hair. It looks glossy, has very little frizz, and rebounds from stretches. Conversely, damaged hair experiences moisture imbalance, protein loss, and cuticle erosion. This causes hair that feels rough to the touch, is readily broken, and is dull, frizzy, and brittle.

Typical reasons for hair damage consist of:

1. Overuse of heat styling
2. Extensive chemical processes (such as perming, bleaching, or dying)
3. Environmental elements (pollution, sun exposure)
4. An inadequate nutrition and thirst

1.2 TYPICAL HAIR ISSUES AND THEIR ROOT CAUSES

Frizz and Dryness

When the scalp doesn't create enough sebum or when outside influences deplete the moisture in the hair, dry hair results. Dryness frequently results in frizz because it raises the hair's cuticle, which makes it easier for airborne moisture to enter and inflate the hair.

Reasons for frizz and dryness:

1. Overdoing hair cleaning, which removes natural oils
2. Using sulfate-containing harsh shampoos
3. Overuse of heat styling tools without proper safety
4. Being outside in dry or humid weather

To fight frizz and dryness:

1. Make use of hydrating shampoos and conditioners without sulfates.
2. Include leave-in conditioners or hair oils in your regimen.

3. usage heat protectant consistently and limit the usage of heat-generating tools.

Scalp Rashes and Dandruff

Unbalanced scalp health, frequently brought on by excessive oil production, dryness, or fungal growth, is the cause of dandruff. It comes in the form of white flakes and may cause discomfort or itching.

Dandruff causes:

1. Overgrowth of Malassezia, a naturally occurring yeast on the scalp
2. Excessive oil production or dry skin
3. Product sensitivity for hair care
4. Infrequent washing, which causes accumulation of oil

To control dandruff:

- Make use of an anti-dandruff shampoo with active components such as ketoconazole or zinc pyrithione.
- Steer clear of too abrasive styling products since

they may irritate the scalp.

- Maintain a clean, moisturized scalp.

Thinning and Hair Loss

Common problems like hair loss and thinning can be brought on by a number of things, including lifestyle choices and heredity. A daily loss of 50-100 hairs is typical, but more than that can be cause for concern.

Reasons for thinning and hair loss:

1. Genetics (alopecia androgenetica)
2. Hormonal shifts, such as menopause and postpartum hair loss
3. Inadequate intake of iron, vitamin D, and protein
4. Stress, disease, or certain drugs

In order to deal with hair loss:

1. Keep up a healthy, vitamin- and mineral-rich diet to support the health of your hair.
2. To encourage hair growth, think about applying

topical treatments like minoxidil.

3. Speak with a medical expert if the issue continues.

Breakage and Split Ends

When the protecting cuticle is lost, the hair strand frays and split ends result. Breakage occurs when the hair weakens and breaks off, usually in the middle or at the ends.

Reasons for breakage and split ends:

1. Abuse of heat styling equipment
2. Regular use of chemicals
3. Tough treatment, such as vigorous brushing or towel drying
4. Damage from the environment, like UV exposure

To avoid breakage and split ends:

1. Regularly trim hair to eliminate damaged ends.
2. Use protective serums and avoid overheating hairstyles.
3. Use a gentle brush or wide-tooth comb to gently

detangle hair.

1.3 SCALP HEALTH: AN ESSENTIAL ASPECT

The Relationship Between Hair Growth and Scalp Health

Hair that is vibrant and strong is built on a healthy scalp. Like the skin on the rest of the body, the scalp need adequate maintenance and nutrition to perform at its best. Poor scalp health, whether it be excessively dry, oily, or inflammatory, has a direct effect on hair growth and quality. Problems with the scalp can lead to clogged follicles, interfere with the hair growth cycle, and result in dandruff, irritation, and even hair loss.

To encourage the growth of healthy hair:

1. Maintain a clean scalp, but avoid over-washing.
2. Regularly massage the scalp to encourage oxygen supply to hair follicles and blood flow.
3. Make use of products made to maintain and replenish the moisture balance of the scalp.

Recognizing Typical Scalp Conditions

Early detection and treatment of scalp issues might stop them from having a detrimental impact on your hair. Among the most typical problems with the scalp are:

- **Seborrheic dermatitis:** A disorder that frequently results in dandruff and causes red, flaky spots on the scalp.

- An autoimmune disease called psoriasis causes thick, scaly skin patches.

- **Folliculitis:** An infection or inflammation of the hair follicles that results in painful red lumps.

- Patchy hair loss is a symptom of the autoimmune disease Alopecia areata.

For appropriate therapy, it is imperative to see a dermatologist if any of these symptoms are present.

Appropriate Methods for Scalp Care

Just as facial skincare calls for particular methods and goods, so too should scalp care be considered carefully:

- **Cleanse:** To get rid of debris, oil, and product buildup, use a mild shampoo without sulfates. Steer clear of really strong washes that may remove natural oils.

- **Exfoliate**: To encourage healthy cell turnover and get rid of dead skin cells, exfoliate your scalp once or twice a month. Seek for exfoliating shampoos or scalp washes that include salicylic acid.

- **Moisturize:** To keep your scalp hydrated if it's dry, use a moisturizing conditioner or serum. Organic oils such as argan or jojoba oil have certain advantages.

- **Massage:** To enhance circulation and promote hair development, include scalp massages in your regimen.

Taking good care of the scalp helps avoid many different hair and scalp problems and guarantees a healthy environment for hair growth.

You can efficiently manage and take care of your hair by being aware of its structure, recognizing frequent issues, and placing a high priority on the health of your scalp. For many years to come, this fundamental understanding will support you in keeping your hair strong, healthy, and attractive.

CHAPTER 2

Natural Ingredients' Power

An increasing trend in recent years has been the inclusion of natural products in routines for both health and beauty. This change isn't just a fad; rather, it's a return to the tried-and-true natural medicines that people from all walks of life have been using for ages. Natural substances have a special power when it comes to hair care because they are typically kinder to the hair and scalp, support general hair health, and support ethical and sustainable activities. This chapter goes into great detail about the advantages of utilizing natural products, the function of essential oils in hair care, and the internal support that superfoods may provide for healthy hair.

2.1 Advantages of Natural Product Use

Steer clear of synthetic ingredients and harsh chemicals

The avoidance of harsh chemicals and synthetic components, which over time can damage the hair and scalp, is one of the main benefits of utilizing natural hair care products. Sulfates, parabens, silicones, and artificial perfumes are present in a lot of commercial hair products, and they can all lead to:

1. **Irritation of the scalp:** Sulfates and other chemicals can deplete the scalp of its natural oils, causing dryness, irritation, and in severe cases, allergic responses.

2. **Weakened hair structure:** Hair's protein structure can be broken down by repeated exposure to synthetic chemicals, increasing the likelihood of breakage and split ends.

3. **Product buildup:** Silicones, which are frequently present in hair products, have the tendency to coat the hair shaft, resulting in buildup that makes hair appear greasy and less shiny.

Conversely, natural products typically don't contain these dangerous substances and offer a more comprehensive approach to hair care. They aid in preserving the proper balance of moisture and general health of the hair by gently cleansing and nourishing it without removing its natural oils.

The Remedies Found in Natural Substances

Natural components are rich in nutrients, antioxidants, and therapeutic qualities that are good for the hair and scalp. Many of these ingredients are derived from plants, flowers, fruits, and herbs. These components, in contrast to their synthetic counterparts, are frequently biocompatible with the body, which means they complement the natural functions of the skin and hair. Principal advantages consist of:

1. **Moisture retention**: To keep the hair shaft from becoming dry and brittle, natural oils like coconut, argan, and jojoba help lock in moisture.
2. **Soother irritation:** Due to their well-known anti-inflammatory and calming qualities, ingredients like chamomile and aloe vera are perfect for sensitive or irritated scalps.
3. **Strengthening:** The hair shaft can be strengthened

by plant proteins, such as those found in rice or quinoa, which lower breakage and promote growth.

The Significance of Ethical Sourcing and Sustainability

The focus on sustainability and ethical sourcing that comes with utilizing natural hair care products is another significant advantage. Conventional beauty products frequently participate in environmentally harmful practices or depend on the extraction of non-renewable resources. Natural goods, especially those with fair trade or certified organic certification, give priority to:

1. **Sustainable harvesting:** Measures to preserve biodiversity and lessen environmental effects are frequently used when sourcing ingredients.
2. **Ethical labor practices:** A lot of natural product companies collaborate directly with cooperatives and small-scale farmers to guarantee that laborers receive fair compensation and treatment.
3. **Reduced carbon footprint:** Natural product manufacturers are more environmentally friendly because they usually don't utilize pesticides,

hazardous chemicals, or a lot of energy.

Customers who choose natural products promote the health of the environment and the people who grow the items, as well as a more sustainable beauty sector.

2.2 HAIR CARE ESSENTIAL OILS

Advantages of Using Essential Oils

Essential oils are highly concentrated extracts with potent components that are good for the health of the hair and scalp. They are made from different parts of plants using techniques like steam distillation or cold pressing. Due to its many advantages, which include the following, their use in hair care has greatly increased:

1. **Stimulating hair growth:** Hair follicles can be nourished and faster, healthier hair growth can be encouraged by essential oils like peppermint and rosemary, which increase blood circulation in the scalp.

2. **Balancing oil production:** Tea tree and lavender

oils are great for people with oily or acne-prone scalps since they help control the natural oil production of the scalp.

3. **Treating scalp issues:** Dandruff, scalp psoriasis, and other common scalp problems can be effectively treated by several essential oils due to their antifungal, antibacterial, and anti-inflammatory qualities.

Well-liked Essential Oils for Healthy Hair Growth

1. Lavender Oil: In addition to having an aroma that is relaxing, lavender oil contains antimicrobial qualities that can help maintain a healthy scalp and stave off dandruff. Additionally, it might lessen stress, which is connected to hair loss.

2. Peppermint Oil: Cooling and energizing, peppermint oil improves blood flow to the scalp. Research has indicated that by reviving the hair follicles, it may promote hair growth.

3. Rosemary Oil: Known to enhance hair thickness and

development by promoting blood circulation, rosemary oil is one of the most often used essential oils for hair. Additionally, it's used to lessen dandruff and premature graying.

4. Tea Tree Oil: Tea tree oil has potent antibacterial and antifungal qualities that can help unclog hair follicles and relieve rashes on the scalp. It works particularly well for dandruff and inflammation of the scalp.

5. Cedarwood Oil: This oil has antifungal qualities and regulates the scalp's oil-producing glands. Cedarwood is frequently used to stop hair loss and encourage the development of new hair.

Safe Use of Essential Oils

Even though essential oils have a lot to give, it's important to use them correctly to prevent any negative consequences. Because of their high concentration, these oils shouldn't be administered topically to the skin or scalp in their undiluted state. Safe use consists of:

- **Dilution:** Almond, coconut, or jojoba oils are excellent choices for dilution when using essential oils. Three to five drops of essential oil are typically added to one tablespoon of carrier oil.

- **Patch test:** To rule out allergic reactions, test a small patch of skin before using any essential oil mixture on your scalp or hair.

- **Massage:** To promote blood flow and guarantee even distribution, gently massage the diluted essential oil combination into the scalp.

- **Avoid overuse:** Moderate use is recommended for essential oils. Overuse can cause irritation, discomfort, or accumulation that can clog hair follicles on the scalp.

2.3 SUPERFOODS THAT PROMOTE HEALTHY HAIR

Superfoods' Nutritious Value

Superfoods are foods that are high in nutrients and contain

a lot of vitamins, minerals, antioxidants, and good fats. These meals are essential for maintaining healthy hair in addition to being good for general health. Keratin, the protein that makes human hair, needs enough nourishment to develop strong and healthily. The appropriate ratio of nutrients can:

1. **Support hair growth:** Zinc, biotin, and vitamin E are among the vitamins and minerals that are necessary for healthy hair growth.

2. **Strengthen hair strands:** The hair shaft is strengthened by the proteins and antioxidants found in superfoods, which lessen breakage and split ends.

3. **Prevent hair loss:** By enhancing circulation and nourishing hair follicles, iron, omega-3 fatty acids, and B vitamins found in superfoods help prevent hair loss.

Superfoods That Encourage Strength and Hair Growth

1. Spinach: Packed with iron, vitamin A, and C, spinach helps keep the scalp healthy and stimulates hair growth by supplying nutrients and oxygen to hair follicles.

2. Sweet Potatoes: Rich in beta-carotene, sweet potatoes aid in the production of sebum, a naturally occurring oil that lubricates the scalp and maintains healthy, lustrous hair.

3. Salmon: Rich in protein, vitamin D, and omega-3 fatty acids, salmon promotes general hair thickness, lowers inflammation, and fortifies hair.

4. Avocados: Packed with antioxidants, vitamin E, and good fats, avocados shield hair from oxidative damage and maintain its strength and hydration.

5. Eggs: A great source of biotin and protein, eggs are essential for healthy hair development. A lack of biotin can cause hair loss or thinning.

Including Superfoods in Your Meal Plan

You may greatly enhance the health of your hair by including these superfoods in your regular diet. Here are some useful examples on how to incorporate them:

1. **Smoothies:** For a quick and simple nutritional boost, blend spinach, avocado, and other nutrient-rich fruits like berries into a smoothie.

2. **Salads:** For a high-protein, hair-strengthening lunch, top your salad with boiled eggs or salmon.

3. **Snacks:** Eat nuts and seeds that are high in vitamins and minerals that are vital for healthy hair, such chia seeds and almonds.

4. **Breakfast:** Indulge in a bowl of oats topped with chia or flax seeds, two superfoods high in omega-3 fatty acids that support good hair development.

Knowing the advantages of natural products, essential oils, and superfoods will help you make well-informed choices regarding your hair care regimen. Accepting the power of nature promotes healthier hair and helps advance a more ethical and sustainable definition of beauty.

CHAPTER 3

Customizing Smoothie Treatments for Hair

Smoothies for hair have become popular as a healthy, natural, and adaptable remedy for a range of hair issues. Nutrient-rich substances can be combined into a mask-like treatment to give your hair a significant health and vibrancy boost. These treatments are simple to prepare, adaptable, and may be customized to meet your unique hair requirements. This chapter will cover the fundamentals of creating hair smoothies, offer solutions for frequent hair issues, and demonstrate how to tailor hair smoothie treatments to your individual hair objectives.

3.1 The Fundamentals of Preparing Hair Smoothies

Selecting Appropriate Ingredients

Choosing the correct components is the cornerstone of every hair smoothie treatment. Each substance has distinct qualities that can help with particular issues including frizz, dryness, inflammation of the scalp, or hair loss. It's crucial to select ingredients for your customized hair smoothie based on the kind and requirements of your hair:

- **Ingredients for moisturizing:** These moisturize parched hair, giving it a smoother, more glossy finish. Aloe vera, avocado, coconut milk, honey, and banana are a few examples.

- **Strengthening substances:** Vitamin and protein-rich compounds are crucial for weak or damaged hair. Oats, Greek yogurt, and eggs are excellent choices for preserving the structure of the hair.

- **Scalp-soothing substances:** Look for anti-inflammatory components like apple cider vinegar, aloe vera, or tea tree oil if you have a sensitive or flaky scalp. These compounds help reduce inflammation and balance the health of your scalp.

- **substances that promote hair growth:** Foods high in biotin, such eggs and almonds, as well as substances like castor oil and rosemary oil help support the health of follicles and promote hair growth.

The selection of each ingredient has to be based on your long-term objectives and existing hair problems. For instance, you might want to concentrate on adding moisturizing elements like banana and honey to seal in moisture if you have dry hair.

Blending Methods for Best Outcomes

For optimal vitamin uptake and even application, a smooth, well-blended smoothie is essential. Here's how to make sure your therapy functions at its optimum and obtain the best consistency:

- **Use a high-speed blender:** Blend all the ingredients well in a blender for the smoothest texture. This guarantees that there are no lumps, which could make it challenging to apply the smoothie to the scalp and hair uniformly.

- **modify liquid content:** You may need to add more or less liquid to modify the consistency, depending on the ingredients used. Use ingredients like avocado or coconut cream for thicker smoothies. Add water, herbal tea, or aloe vera juice to thin the mixture.

- **Avoid over-blending:** Although thorough blending is crucial, excessive bleeding may cause some proteins and vitamins in fragile ingredients, such as fruits or oils, to be broken down and lose some of their potency. Blend just till creamy and smooth.

Using Hair Smoothies to Treat Your Hair and Scalp

After blending your smoothie, it's time to apply it correctly to get the most out of it:

- **Section your hair:** To guarantee that the smoothie is dispersed evenly, begin by dividing your hair into manageable portions. For hair types that are curly or thick, this is quite crucial.

- **Massage into the scalp:** Apply the smoothie straight to your scalp using your fingers. In addition to helping to get nutrients straight to the hair follicles, this increases blood circulation.

- **Pay attention to the ends:** Usually, the driest and most damaged sections of the hair are the ends. Make sure to apply a thick layer of coating to avoid breakage and broken ends.

- **Leave on for 20–30 minutes**: To ensure the ingredients absorb completely, wrap your hair in a warm towel or shower cap after application. Your hair's cuticles will open up from the heat, improving absorption.

- **Completely rinse:** Use lukewarm water to rinse the smoothie out of your hair, making sure to get rid of all of the product. If necessary, proceed with a mild shampoo and end with a conditioner.

3.2 Hair Smoothie Formulas for Typical Issues

Frizzed Out and Dry Hair

A highly hydrating smoothie can help restore moisture balance to dry, brittle, or frizzy hair, leaving it lustrous and silky. Rich softeners and moisturizers are combined in this recipe:

Components:

1. One ripe avocado
2. Two tablespoons of coconut milk - One tablespoon of honey
3. One banana

- **Avocado and coconut milk** give intense moisture and smooth the hair shaft, which are two of the benefits.
- Honey draws moisture into the hair by acting as a natural humectant.
- Banana infuses potassium and vitamins into the hair, softening and improving manageability.

Application: Work the smoothie into the driest areas of the body, working your way up from the roots. After 30 minutes, leave it on and give it a thorough rinse.

Scalp Rashes and Dandruff

Dandruff can be treated, and an inflamed scalp can be soothed, with the aid of an antibacterial hair smoothie. Anti-inflammatory and balancing substances are combined in this recipe:

Components:

1. One tablespoon apple cider vinegar
2. two tablespoons aloe vera gel
3. three drops tea tree oil
4. one tablespoon honey

Benefits:

1. Aloe vera moisturizes and relieves irritation of the scalp.
2. Apple cider vinegar lowers flakiness and restores pH balance to the scalp.
3. The antifungal qualities of tea tree oil help fight

infection and dandruff.

4. Honey helps seal in moisture and lessen inflammation.

Apply: Apply the smoothie directly to the scalp and roots, massage, and then rinse with a mild shampoo after 20 minutes.

Thinning and Hair Loss

In order to achieve fuller, healthier hair, this hair smoothie is meant to fortify the roots, encourage hair development, and nourish the follicles:

Components:

1. One protein-rich egg, one tablespoon castor oil, and one teaspoon essential rosemary oil

2. Two tsp Greek yogurt

Advantages:
Product:

1. Egg offers vital protein to fortify hair.

2. Castor oil thickens thinning hair and promotes hair

growth.

3. **Essential rosemary oil** improves circulation to the scalp, encouraging the creation of new hair.

4. **Greek yogurt** is high in lactic acid and protein, which helps to exfoliate the scalp and promote hair development.

Application: Massage your scalp thoroughly after applying this smoothie. After 30 minutes, let it sit and then rinse with cool water.

Breakage and Split Ends

A nourishing hair smoothie can supply the essential proteins and moisture to repair and shield damaged hair that is prone to breakage and split ends:

Components:

1. One tablespoon of coconut oil - Two tablespoons of powdered oatmeal

2. Two tablespoons of aloe vera juice - One spoonful of honey

Advantages:

1. Protein loss is strengthened and avoided by coconut oil.

2. Oatmeal relieves irritated scalps and restores the hair shaft.

3. Honey aids in keeping moisture in the hair to stop more damage.

4. Juice of aloe vera replenishes and strengthens damaged endings.

Application: If your scalp is greasy, concentrate the smoothie on the mid-lengths and ends of your hair. After 20 minutes, remove with lukewarm water and rinse.

3.3 Customizing Your Smoothie Treatments

Determining Your Particular Hair Needs

Identifying your individual hair difficulties and assessing your hair type is the first step towards personalizing your hair smoothie treatment. Considerable elements include:

- **Hair texture:** Is it curly, straight, coarse, or fine?

Varied amounts of moisture and protein are needed for varied textures.

- **Hair porosity:** While low-porosity hair can find it difficult to absorb cosmetics, once sealed, it keeps moisture. High-porosity hair absorbs moisture quickly but also loses it quickly.

- **Scalp condition:** If you have an oily scalp, look for components that are lighter and more clarifying. Use moisturizing and nourishing ingredients for dry scalps.

You may more effectively customize your smoothies to your hair's particular requirements by being aware of its special qualities.

Using Your Preferred Ingredients

The ability to include your preferred ingredients based on your experiences and tastes is one benefit of creating your own hair smoothies. You can use items that you adore for their taste, texture, or special qualities. Here are some pointers:

- **Herbs:** Include dried or fresh herbs, such as hibiscus, basil, or rosemary, as they are proven to improve the health and growth of hair.

- **Essential oils:** Customize your smoothie by adding essential oils that are appropriate for your hair and scalp. For example, peppermint and lavender oils are great for energizing and relaxing the scalp.

- **Superfoods:** Antioxidants and nutrients that support overall hair health may be found in ingredients like spirulina, matcha, and chia seeds, which can give your hair smoothie an extra nutritional boost.

Testing Out Various Combinations

Making your own hair smoothies gives you the freedom to try out different ingredient combinations and see which ones work best for your hair. You can modify the recipes over time to account for shifting hair needs, phases of hair development, and seasonal variations. Among the concepts for testing are:

- **Seasonal adjustments:** Use lighter components like cucumber and green tea to assist regulate oil production in the summer, and moisturizing ingredients like aloe vera and coconut milk during the dry winter months.

- **Treating evolving hair needs:** You can adjust the ingredients in your smoothies based on how your hair grows or changes as a result of aging, hormone changes, or environmental influences.

Making customized hair smoothies is a powerful method to take charge of the health of your hair. By being aware of the fundamental methods, utilizing specific formulas, and

By tailoring your treatments, you can use natural, nutrient-rich products to get hair that is stronger, healthier, and more bright.

CHAPTER 4

OPTIMAL OUTCOMES WITH HAIR CARE ROUTINES

It takes more than simply the correct products to achieve and maintain healthy hair; it also takes a regular regimen that supports hair health and attends to individual demands. Over time, a comprehensive hair care regimen can assist you in achieving the best results possible, regardless of the type of hair you have—dry, frizzy, greasy, or damaged. The fundamentals of a thorough hair care routine, from cleansing and conditioning to deep treatments and delicate styling methods, will be covered in detail in this chapter.

4.1 HAIR WASHING AND CONDITIONING

How Often Should You Wash?

Numerous factors, such as hair type, scalp health, and lifestyle, influence how often you wash your hair. Knowing when to wash your hair is essential to keeping the ratio of hydration to cleanliness in check.

Hair Type:

1. Oily hair has a propensity to rapidly build up sebum, which can result in greasy roots. Maintaining a clean scalp may require washing three to four times a week.

2. On the other hand, dry or curly hair might benefit from washing 1-2 times a week less frequently to prevent removing natural oils that are essential for hydration.

3. Normal hair types may strike a balance by washing 2-3 times a week or every other day, contingent on environmental conditions such as physical activity or pollutants.

Scalp Condition: Those with sensitive or dry scalps should try to wash less frequently to avoid irritation, while those with dandruff or scalp disorders like psoriasis may need to wash more regularly with specific solutions.

Lifestyle: While people in colder climates or with less exposure to environmental toxins can wash less frequently, active people who exercise frequently and perspire more may need to wash more frequently to keep their scalp clean.

Selecting the Appropriate Shampoo and Conditioner

Maintaining healthy, manageable hair requires choosing the right shampoo and conditioner based on your hair type and issues.

1. **Shampoo**: Shampoo's main purpose is to wash the scalp and get rid of debris, oil, and product buildup. Choose a shampoo based on your unique requirements:
2. Although clarifying shampoos can strip hair of essential oils, they should only be used sparingly to thoroughly clean and get rid of buildup and excess oil.
3. Hydrating or moisturizing shampoos are great for dry or curly hair because they add moisture without making the hair feel heavy.
4. Volumizing shampoos remove oil that may weigh down the strands of hair gently, lifting fine or flat

hair.

5. Sulfate-free shampoos are the best choice for people with color-treated hair or sensitive scalps because they don't include harsh chemicals that might irritate skin or bleed color.

Conditioner: Conditioner adds hydration, smoothes the cuticle of hair, and lessens frizz. The same as shampoo, choose the correct conditioner is essential:

1. Lightweight conditioners hydrate hair without making it greasy, making them perfect for fine or oily hair.
2. Rich, hydrating elements included in deep conditioners help to restore the strength and flexibility of dry or damaged hair.
3. Leave-in conditioners provide further detangling and frizz control and are great for adding extra hydration throughout the day.

Appropriate Cleaning and Conditioning Methods

The methods you employ when washing and conditioning your hair, even with the best products, are quite important to keeping it healthy. The following are some recommended procedures:

Washing:

1. Use lukewarm water to completely soak your hair at first, since hot water might dry out your scalp and hair.
2. Apply a small amount of shampoo to the scalp and lather it between your palms. Use your fingertips, not your nails, gently massage the scalp in order to promote circulation and eliminate accumulation.
3. Refrain from vigorously massaging the length of your hair as this may cause breaking and tangling.
4. Make sure to fully rinse away all of the product.

Conditioning:

1. Since the ends of the hair sustain the most damage, concentrate your conditioner application there. Unless your hair is extremely dry, try not to use too much conditioner at the roots of your hair.
2. Use a wide-tooth comb to thoroughly and evenly spread the conditioner.
3. To seal the hair cuticle and add shine and

smoothness, let the conditioner rest for a few minutes to allow for proper absorption before washing with cool water.

4.2 Hair masks and deep conditioners

Deep Conditioning's Advantages

Any hair care regimen must include deep conditioning, but it's especially important for those whose hair is dry, damaged, or has had chemical treatment. Deep conditioners and hair masks, in contrast to ordinary conditioners, penetrate the hair shaft more deeply and offer intense hydration and nourishment.

- **Hydration:** Deep conditioning treatments are particularly helpful for dry, curly, or coily hair types that have trouble holding onto moisture since they help restore lost moisture.

- **Strengthening:** Over time, breakage and split ends are lessened by the proteins that deep conditioners frequently contain to help mend weak or damaged hair.

- **Improving suppleness:** Regular deep conditioning helps increase the suppleness of the hair, making it more resistant to stretching and style and lowering the risk of breakage.

DIY Deep Conditioning Procedures

Handmade deep conditioners make a great alternative for individuals looking for something affordable and natural. These treatments offer individualized solutions based on your unique demands and frequently make use of common kitchen items.

Olive Oil and Avocado Mask: This mask adds luster and deeply hydrates dry, brittle hair thanks to its rich content of important fatty acids and vitamins.

- **Components:** 2 tablespoons of olive oil and one ripe avocado
- **Instructions:** Smoothly blend the oil and avocado together. Apply to wet hair, paying special attention to the ends, and let sit for half an hour before

washing.

Honey and Coconut Milk Mask: Coconut milk fortifies and repairs hair, while honey, a natural humectant, attracts moisture into the strands.

- **Components:** Three tablespoons coconut milk and two tablespoons honey
- **Instructions:** Combine the ingredients and use on damp, clean hair. After 20 minutes, remove with lukewarm water and rinse.

How to Put on and Take Off Hair Masks

The following application and cleaning methods must be followed to get the most out of hair masks and deep conditioners:

Application:

1. To ensure optimal absorption, apply deep conditioners or masks only to moist, clean hair. Product buildup may impede this process.
2. Apply the product evenly using your fingers or a wide-tooth comb, being especially careful around the

ends where damage is most likely to occur.

Rinsing:

1. Wear the mask for the suggested amount of time, usually 20 to 30 minutes. You can apply a shower cap or wrap your hair in a warm towel to generate heat for deeper hydration. This will allow the product to seep into your hair more thoroughly.

2. Rinse with cool water to seal the cuticle of the hair and retain moisture, making sure all product is completely gone to prevent residue.

4.3 GENTLY STYLE YOUR HAIR

Steer clear of heat styling whenever you can

Over time, heat style can seriously harm hair, resulting in split ends, dryness, and even hair loss. Although heat styling appliances like curling irons, blow dryers, and straighteners are convenient, using them less often will preserve the integrity of your hair.

- **Embrace Air Drying:** Let your hair air dry

naturally whenever you can. Use a microfiber towel or t-shirt to gently pat your hair after washing to absorb extra water and lessen friction, which can cause frizz.

- **Heat-Free Styling Techniques:** There are numerous methods for styling hair without the use of heat. While hair rollers can give volume or curls without the need for a curling iron, braiding damp hair can produce natural waves. Furthermore, adding texture or defining curls can be achieved by using style creams or mousses to damp hair.

Applying Heat Shielding When Required

Using a heat protectant is essential to reduce damage if heat styling cannot be avoided. By erecting a barrier between your hair and the heat, heat protectants help to keep moisture in and shield the hair cuticle from direct heat exposure.

- Selecting the Appropriate Heat Protectant: Choose a heat protectant based on the type of hair you have and the tool's temperature. Richer creams or serums are best for thick or coarse hair, while lightweight sprays are great for fine hair.

- **Apply Correctly:** Distribute the heat protectant evenly throughout your hair, paying special attention to the ends and mid-lengths, which are the areas most vulnerable to damage. To prevent burning your hair, wait until your hair is totally dry before using any heated tools.

Soft Styling Methods

By including mild style techniques into your routine, you can lessen the chance of breakage and split ends by giving your hair less needless stress. The following advice can help you style your hair while maintaining its health:

- **Use a Wide-Tooth Comb:** After washing, detangle wet hair (which is more brittle and prone to breaking than dried hair) using a wide-tooth comb. To prevent undue strain on the roots, begin at the ends and work your way up.

- **Select Loose Hairstyles:** Tight braids, buns, and ponytails can strain the hair, causing breakage and perhaps even hair loss. Choose looser haircuts that won't strain the hair shaft or scalp.

- **Make the Switch to Silk or Satin:** Use hair ties and silk or satin pillowcases to lessen friction, which will stop breaking and frizz. Elastic hair ties can produce dents and weaken the hair, while cotton pillowcases can lead to tangles and breakage.

- **Regular Trims:** Keeping your hair healthy requires regular trims. Trimming your hair every 6 to 8 weeks will help prevent split ends, maintain the health of your hair, and encourage smoother growth even if you're aiming to grow it long.

An all-encompassing hair care regimen can make all the distinction in terms of having vibrant, healthy hair. You can preserve your hair and bring out its inherent beauty by using gentle styling techniques, adding deep conditioning treatments, and selecting high-quality products.

CHAPTER 5

MAINTENANCE AND GROWTH OF HAIR

Achieving and sustaining healthy hair growth is a journey that includes taking care of your scalp, adopting habits that encourage strength and longevity, and tending to your hair from the roots up. This chapter will cover techniques for promoting hair development, preserving length and thickness, and customizing care regimens for various hair types. Making the correct lifestyle choices and hair care practices is essential if you want to retain healthy hair, thicken thinning areas, or grow long hair.

5.1 HAIR GROWTH STIMULATION

Numerous factors, such as diet, lifestyle choices, scalp health, and heredity, affect hair development. It's critical to prioritize both outward care and interior wellness in order to promote optimal growth.

The Advantages of Scalp Massages

Regular scalp massages are among the easiest and most efficient ways to promote hair development. By promoting blood circulation, scalp massage helps the hair follicles receive vital nutrients. This stimulation might improve the environment on the scalp and stimulate hair growth.

- **Improved Circulation:** By increasing blood flow to the hair follicles, scalp massages aid in giving them the nutrients and oxygen necessary for growth.

- **Reduction of Stress and Relaxation:** It is well known that stress can impede the growth of hair. Frequent scalp massages not only promote development but also aid in lowering stress, which might lessen the possibility of tension-related hair loss.

- **Application Techniques:** Every day, spend five to ten minutes using your fingertips to gently massage the scalp in circular patterns. Use organic oils such as castor, coconut, or argan to fortify the roots of your hair and nourish your scalp even more.

Hair Growth Supplements: An Analysis of Their Potency

The purpose of hair growth supplements is to supply the body with the vitamins and minerals necessary for normal, healthy hair development. Even though some supplements have been shown to provide benefits, each person's health and hair conditions can affect how helpful a supplement is.

- **Vitamin B7, biotin:** Biotin, well-known for supporting healthy skin, hair, and nails, aids in strengthening hair and halting thinning. The protein known as keratin, which comprises hair strands, is produced with its assistance.

- **Vitamin D:** Hair loss has been connected to vitamin D deficiency. Supplements that stimulate dormant hair follicles can aid in stimulating hair growth.

- **Iron:** One of the most frequent reasons for hair loss, especially in women, is an iron deficiency. Iron supplements help reestablish the equilibrium required for healthy hair development.

- **Zinc:** Zinc promotes tissue regeneration and helps control sebum production, both of which are essential for normal hair development on the scalp.

Speak with your doctor before beginning any supplement regimen to find out if it's required and to make sure it's safe given your particular medical circumstances.

Encouraging Internal Hair Growth

The foundation of healthy hair is within. Your food is a major factor in giving your body the nutrition it needs to maintain hair growth. Your hair can become healthier overall if you incorporate a diet high in vitamins, minerals, and proteins that is well-balanced.

- **Foods High in Protein:** Keratin, a kind of protein, is the main component of hair. Eating foods high in protein, such as fish, eggs, lean meats, nuts, and legumes, can strengthen the structure of hair and keep it from becoming brittle.

- **Healthy Fats:** By lowering inflammation and supplying important oils to the hair, omega-3 fatty acids, which are present in walnuts, flaxseeds, and fish, help enhance scalp health.

- **Hydration:** Maintaining healthy hair requires your body to be well hydrated. By keeping your hair moisturized from the inside out, drinking adequate water helps shield it from drying out and breaking.

- **Antioxidants and Vitamins:** Vitamins A, C, and E-rich leafy greens, berries, and fruits protect hair follicles from oxidative stress and increase the synthesis of natural oils that moisturize the scalp.

5.2 PRESERVING HAIR THICKNESS AND LENGTH

Once your hair begins to grow, it's critical to preserve its length and thickness. This entails forming habits that reduce damage, stop breakage, and maintain the health of your hair over time.

Consistent Trimming for Healthier Ends

While it may seem counterproductive to routinely trim your hair when trying to grow it longer, doing so is necessary to preserve healthy ends. As damaged hair and split ends move up the hair shaft, further breaking may eventually occur.

- **Benefits of Regular Trims:** Regular trims assist get rid of split ends before they cause serious harm. Trimming should occur every 6 to 8 weeks. This maintains the appearance of healthier, smoother, and fuller hair.

- **Length Retention:** Regular trims help to prevent excessive breakage, which eventually enables you to keep length more effectively, even if you may lose some length with each trim.

Avoiding Breakage and Split Ends

Your hair's length and thickness can be preserved by

avoiding split ends and breaking. You can reduce the harm that regular styling and environmental variables inflict by implementing preventative steps.

- **Moisturization:** One of the finest strategies to stop breaking is to keep your hair well-hydrated. Use hair oils or leave-in conditioners on a frequent basis because dry hair is more prone to breaking and splitting.

- **Avoiding Overuse of Heat:** Split ends and breakage can result from heat styling weakening the hair cuticle. When utilizing hot tools, wear a heat protectant at all times or use as little as possible of blow dryers, curling wands, and flat irons.

- **Gentle Detangling:** To prevent tugging and breaking, disentangle wet hair using a wide-tooth comb or your fingers, working your way up from the ends.

Preventing Damage to Your Hair

For your hair to stay healthy and thick, frequent trimming and moisturizing are essential, but so is shielding it from the elements.

- **Environmental Protection:** Harsh weather, pollutants, and UV radiation can seriously harm hair. When spending a lot of time outside, use a UV protection spray or wear a hat.

- **Protective Hairstyles:** If you have longer or textured hair, wearing your hair in protective styles like braids, twists, or buns can help reduce everyday styling wear and tear.

- **Nighttime Protection:** Using satin or silk pillows lessens the chance of breakage and tangles in your hair while you sleep. Moreover, a silk or satin scarf can assist retain moisture in your hair.

5.3 Hair Type-Specific Hair Care Advice

Every hair type is different and needs different care practices to maintain, grow, and look their best. Creating a hair care routine that works for your specific hair type requires an understanding of its requirements.

Care Advice for Curly Hair

Because of the way that curly hair is shaped, it is more likely to be dry and frizzy, which hinders natural oils from getting from the scalp to the ends of the hair. Curly hair therefore needs more moisture and careful attention.

- **Moisturizing Routine:** Use moisturizing conditioners and shampoos without sulfates to prevent your hair from losing its natural oils. To seal in moisture and define curls, use curl creams or leave-in conditioners afterward.

- **Detangling:** To prevent breakage, detangle damp curly hair with your fingers or a wide-tooth comb. To provide slip, detangle in portions using conditioner or a detangling product.

- **Avoid Heat:** Try not to use too much heat styling to avoid destroying the curl pattern. You can keep your natural curls without frizz by air-drying them or using a diffuser on low heat.

Care Advice for Straight Hair

Because natural oils from the scalp may easily move down the hair shaft, straight hair tends to grow greasy more quickly. Regular washing and light-weight products that don't weigh the hair down are beneficial for this type of hair.

- **Regular Washing:** To avoid oil accumulation, wash straight hair more regularly (every two to three days). Once a week, use a clarifying shampoo to get rid of any product residue that can build up.

- **Volumizing Products:** Flat hair can occasionally look like straight hair. Use gentle volumizing mousses or sprays, paying special attention to the roots, to increase volume.

- **Protect from Heat:** Apply a heat protectant before blow drying or flat ironing straight hair since it is more vulnerable to heat damage.

Attention to Fine Hair

Having fine hair makes it more brittle and prone to breaking. Heavy items can also cause it to become unwieldy, thus preserving strength and volume calls for a balanced strategy.

- **Lightweight Products:** Opt for fine-hair specific shampoos and conditioners that hydrate hair without making it feel heavy. Products that thicken or volumize hair can make it appear fuller.

- **Strengthening Treatments:** Protein treatments for fine hair can help to strengthen the hair shaft and lessen the chance of breakage.

Refrain from Over-style: Excessive manipulation or overuse of style products can make fine hair appear lifeless. Use mild styling creams or serums instead of thick oils and gels.

You can attain healthy, resilient hair by knowing how to promote hair development, preserve hair length and thickness, and modify your care regimen to fit your particular hair type. By using the proper procedures and maintaining consistency, you can promote your hair's potential for growth and long-term health in addition to improving its appearance.

CHAPTER 6

TREATMENTS FOR HAIR LOSS

For many people, hair loss is a prevalent worry that affects both men and women at different stages of life. People can better manage hair loss by learning the underlying reason of the disease and looking into a variety of alternatives, including both medication and natural therapies. This chapter offers a thorough examination of the many forms and reasons for hair loss, along with the best current cures and treatments.

6.1 KNOWING ABOUT HAIR LOSS

There are many different causes of hair loss, and each person experiences it differently. Understanding the kind and cause of hair loss is the first step in treating it, since this will assist in determining the most effective course of treatment.

Types of Loss of Hair

Hair loss comes in a variety of forms, each with special traits. To appropriately manage your hair loss, you must identify the type of loss you're experiencing:

- **Male or Female Pattern Baldness, or Androgenetic Alopecia:** This is the most prevalent type of hair loss, which frequently runs in the family. It usually shows up as general thinning across the scalp in women, but it usually shows up as a receding hairline and thinning at the crown in men.

- **Alopecia Areata:** Patchy hair loss results from the immune system attacking hair follicles inadvertently. This is not limited to the scalp; it can happen elsewhere on the body and happen unexpectedly.

- **Telogen Effluvium:** This disorder, which is frequently brought on by stress, disease, or hormonal fluctuations, results in a significant number of hair follicles entering the resting phase and widespread thinning.

- **Traction Alopecia:** Tight hairstyles like braids, ponytails, or hair extensions can put physical strain on the hair follicles, resulting in hair loss.

- **Cicatricial (Scarring) Alopecia:** An uncommon ailment that causes inflammation to harm hair follicles and result in irreversible hair loss. In the absence of surgery, scarring frequently happens and the loss is irreparable.

Reasons Behind Hair Loss

A number of reasons, broadly classified as hereditary, environmental, or lifestyle-related, can be linked to hair loss.

- **Genetics:** In many cases of hair loss, especially androgenetic alopecia, heredity plays a significant role. You are more prone to experience hair thinning and eventually loss if baldness runs in your family.

- **Hormonal Changes:** The condition of your hair is greatly influenced by hormones. Hair loss can result from illnesses including menopause, pregnancy, thyroid issues, or hormonal imbalances.

- **Stress and Illness:** Stress, both mental and physical, can cause telogen effluvium by interfering with the hair development cycle. In a similar vein, disease and infections particularly those that impact the scalp may be a factor in hair loss.

- **Deficiencies in Nutrients:** The health of your hair can be adversely affected by a deficiency of certain nutrients, including iron, biotin, and vitamins D and E. Inadequate nourishment debilitates the hair follicles, increasing the likelihood of hair breakage and thinning.

- **Medications and Treatments:** Hair loss can be a side effect of some medications, which include those for high blood pressure, cancer, arthritis, depression, and heart issues. It is also known that chemotherapy and radiation therapy might result in transient hair loss.

- **Hairstyling and Treatments:** If left untreated, traction alopecia, which weakens hair and can become permanent, can be brought on by frequent use of heat styling equipment, chemical treatments, and tight hairstyles.

When to Get Expert Assistance

It's critical to understand when medical intervention is necessary for hair loss. While the occasional shedding of hair is natural, sudden or significant hair loss may indicate a medical problem.

Indications to Look Out For:

1. Abrupt or uneven hair loss
2. Thinning or bald patches
3. Rashes, discomfort, or blisters on the scalp
4. Clumps of hair falling out

It is advised that you see a dermatologist or trichologist who specializes in the care of the hair and scalp if you observe any of these symptoms. Early detection may help treatments work better and perhaps stop hair loss.

6.2 HAIR LOSS NATURAL TREATMENTS

A number of natural treatments have demonstrated potential in lowering shedding and encouraging regeneration for people who favor a more all-encompassing approach to treating hair loss. These treatments can support other therapies and are frequently mild and secure.

Natural Hair Loss Treatments

Traditional medicine has been treating hair loss and thinning for ages using herbal medicines. Among the most widely used herbs are:

- **Saw Palmetto:** Saw palmetto functions by inhibiting the enzyme that converts testosterone into DHT, the hormone associated with hair loss. It is frequently used to treat androgenetic alopecia.

- **Aloe Vera:** Known for its calming qualities, aloe vera aids in reducing irritation in the scalp and fosters a favorable environment for hair development.

- **Rosemary Oil:** It is said that this essential oil may enhance circulation to the scalp and stimulate hair follicles, which may promote hair growth.

- **Green Tea:** Rich in antioxidants, green tea can stop the formation of DHT, which in turn can stop hair loss. While some drink it as part of their daily regimen, others use it as a topical rinse.

Nutritional Adjustments to Encourage Hair Growth

The health of your hair is greatly influenced by what you consume. Making sure your diet is high in proteins, vitamins, and minerals can help to prevent hair loss and encourage hair growth.

- **Foods High in Iron:** Hair loss is frequently caused by low iron levels, especially in women. Iron levels can be raised and hair growth can be encouraged by including foods like spinach, lentils, and lean meats in your diet.

- **Omega-3 Fatty Acids**: Rich in flaxseeds, walnuts, and fatty fish like salmon, omega-3s nourish the hair and scalp while lowering inflammation, which can exacerbate hair loss.

- **Biotin and Zinc:** These two nutrients are vital for healthy, strong hair. They may be found in abundance in eggs, nuts, and seeds.

- **Vitamin D:** Adequate vitamin D levels are essential for healthy hair follicles and can be achieved by sunlight exposure and meals such as fortified dairy, mushrooms, and fatty fish.

Modifications to Lifestyle to Prevent Hair Loss

Modest lifestyle adjustments can make a significant difference in lowering hair loss and enhancing general hair health.

- **Stress Management:** It's critical to develop effective strategies for managing stress because it can exacerbate hair loss. Regular exercise, yoga, and meditation are among techniques that might help lower stress and encourage healthier hair.

- **Gentle Hair Care:** Consider the way you treat your hair every day. To prevent stripping your hair of its natural oils, use sulfate-free shampoos instead of harsh brushes and heat styling products as little as possible.

- **Scalp Care:** Hair development depends on a healthy scalp. Frequent massages of the scalp with oils such as castor or coconut oil will help to maintain healthy follicles and increase blood circulation.

6.3 MEDICAL HAIR LOSS TREATMENTS

Medical therapies can be helpful when natural remedies are insufficient or hair loss is more severe. Surgical procedures and topical treatments are available, based on the needs of the patient and the degree of hair loss.

Medication Prescriptions

For the treatment of hair loss, a number of prescription drugs are available; several of these have undergone clinical testing and received official medical approval.

- **Rogaine, minoxidil:** A common over-the-counter treatment for androgenetic alopecia in both men and women is this topical medication. By boosting blood flow to the scalp and widening hair follicles, minoxidil can stimulate hair growth.

- **Propecia, finasteride):** Finasteride is an oral prescription drug for males that works by lowering the hormone DHT production, which causes male pattern baldness. It is commonly used to treat androgenetic alopecia, and its effectiveness in reducing hair loss and promoting regrowth has been demonstrated.

- **Spironolactone:** A diuretic that also inhibits the

effects of androgens, or male hormones, on the hair follicles, spironolactone is frequently administered to women who are experiencing hormonal hair loss.

Hair Replacement

Hair transplants may be a successful, long-term treatment for people with more severe hair loss. Hair follicles from a healthy part of the scalp (typically the back or sides) are moved to the balding or thinning areas during this surgical treatment.

- **Follicular Unit Transplantation (FUT):** This technique involves removing a strip of scalp, harvesting hair follicles, and transplanting them to the areas that are balding. This method enables more grafts to be done in a single session, although it produces a linear scar.

- **Follicular Unit Extraction (FUE):** FUE is a more recent procedure that involves the removal and transplantation of individual hair follicles to the desired location. Less scarring results from it, and recovery times are shortened, although fewer grafts can be placed in a single session.

Additional Medical Choices

Advanced therapies are becoming more and more popular as additional medical treatments for hair loss because of their ability to effectively stimulate hair regrowth.

- **Platelet-Rich Plasma (PRP) Therapy:** an injection of platelet-rich plasma into the scalp follows the extraction of a patient's blood, which is then processed to concentrate the platelets. This process, which is especially beneficial for people with thinning hair, stimulates hair follicles and promotes regrowth.

- **Low-Level Laser Therapy (LLLT):** LLLT stimulates hair follicles and promotes regrowth by using red light wavelengths. Laser combs and caps are examples of at-home devices that can be used in a clinical environment for this non-invasive treatment.

- **Microneedling:** This technique makes tiny punctures in the scalp with tiny needles. When paired with topical therapies like minoxidil, the technique can improve hair density and thickness by inducing the body's natural healing response.

In order to manage and overcome hair loss, it can be very helpful to understand the sort of hair loss you're experiencing as well as the various therapies and treatments.

Healthy hair development requires a thorough strategy catered to your specific demands, whether you prefer natural remedies or medical procedures.

CHAPTER 7

MEN'S HAIR CARE

Men's hair care has changed dramatically as people have become more conscious of the value of keeping their hair healthy and looking presentable. Even though many men deal with typical hair-related problems like baldness, thinning hair, and scalp diseases, many of these difficulties can be resolved with adequate care. This chapter explores the particulars of hair care for males, covering typical hair issues, styling tips, and practical hair loss remedies.

7.1 TYPICAL MALE HAIR ISSUES

Men have unique hair care needs that are frequently caused by a combination of environmental and hereditary factors. Recognizing these typical problems is the first step toward treating and avoiding additional hair troubles.

Hair Thinning and Baldness

Male Pattern Baldness, also known as Androgenetic Alopecia, is a prevalent hair disorder in men. Usually, it starts as a receding hairline and crown thinning, which can eventually result in partial or total baldness. This mostly inherited illness is brought on by a sensitivity to the hormone dihydrotestosterone (DHT), which causes hair follicles to shrink.

Indicators to Look Out for:

1. Gradual hairline receding (particularly in a "M" shape)
2. Gradual thinning on top of the head
3. Spotty baldness or a more uniform thinning of the scalp

Stress, food, or medical disorders can also cause other types of hair thinning, like telogen effluvium, which causes hair to enter the resting phase too soon and causes extensive shedding.

Beard Maintenance and Care

Men's grooming regimens now heavily incorporate facial hair. Like scalp hair, proper beard maintenance involves routine attention to preserve its health and attractiveness. Men frequently experience the following problems with facial hair:

- **Patchiness:** A man's facial hair may grow thinner in certain places and thicker in others due to uneven beard development.

- **Dryness and Irritation:** If the skin beneath the beard is not adequately moisturized, it may become dry and flaky. Beard hair is frequently coarser than scalp hair.

- **Ingrown Hairs:** These can cause discomfort, rashes, or even infection since hair grows back into the skin rather than outward.

Scalp Health Problems

Hair growth and general health depend on maintaining a healthy scalp. For men, common scalp problems include:

- **Dandruff (Seborrheic Dermatitis):** Dandruff, which is frequently seen as white or yellow flakes, is a result of a flaky scalp brought on by dryness, excessive oil production, or yeast overgrowth.

- **Scalp Psoriasis:** This is a long-term skin disorder that causes red, scaly patches on the scalp. Severe cases can also result in hair loss and itching.

- **Folliculitis:** An inflammation of the hair follicles, frequently brought on by fungi or bacteria, can result in red, inflamed lumps and, in certain situations, hair loss.

7.2 MALE HAIR CARE ADVICE

Even while hair care can appear hard, males can gain from developing easy-to-follow grooming routines. Whether you have facial hair, thinning hair, or a full head of hair, maintaining the health and appearance of your hair will be easier if you use the appropriate products and follow the right procedures.

Men's Grooming Methods

- **Shampooing:** Depending on your hair type and preferences, the number of times you wash depends on how often you shampoo. A mild, sulfate-free shampoo should be used two to three times a week to maintain your scalp clean and avoid dryness.

- **Conditioning:** Although men tend to neglect this process, conditioner is crucial for hydrating hair and avoiding damage. After every wash, use conditioner, paying special attention to the ends of the hair to prevent dragging the scalp down.

- **Brushing and Combing:** To detangle hair, especially while it's damp, use a soft brush or a wide-toothed comb. This reduces the possibility of breaking. A specialist beard comb or brush helps disperse oils and maintains the neat appearance of facial hair.

- **Trimming:** Maintain a well-groomed appearance and avoid split ends with routine trims every 6–8 weeks. Trimming beards helps keep them in form and gets rid of damaged or unkempt hair.

Hair Products Suggestions for Men

Men's hair care products must take into account their particular hair types and problems. The health of your hair and the way it styles can be greatly enhanced by using the correct product.

Shampoos and Conditioners:

1. **Shampoo:** Pick a shampoo suited to your hair type, such as moisturizing for dry hair, clarifying for oily hair, or thickening for thinning hair.

2. **Conditioner:** For coarse or curly hair, go for richer, more hydrating conditioners; for fine hair, go for lighter alternatives.

Styling Products:

1. **Pomade:** Perfect for shorter styles and control, pomades are great for anyone looking for a smooth, glossy finish.

2. **Clay:** Clay products provide volume without making hair look greasy, which is ideal for men with fine or thinning hair who want a matte, textured look.

3. **Hair Wax:** Offers a natural finish with a medium hold, making it appropriate for a variety of everyday styling.

Products for Beard Care:

1. **Oil for Beards:** Preserves skin hydration and beard suppleness. Seek for oils that have coconut, argan, or jojoba oil in them.

2. **Beard Balm:** Helps shape and style longer beards and offers better grip than oil.

3. **Beard Wash and Conditioner:** To keep beard hair supple, use a dedicated beard wash and condition on a regular basis.

Keeping Your Hair and Scalp Healthy

It takes constant attention and care to maintain the health of the hair and scalp. Maintaining healthy hair and avoiding common scalp disorders can be greatly impacted by small behaviors.

- **Avoiding Over-Washing:** Too much shampooing can remove the scalp's natural oils, which can cause dryness or an excessive sebum production. The key is balance.

- **Scalp Exfoliation**: Your scalp can benefit from exfoliation in the same way that your face's skin can. Once a week, use a mild brush or a scalp scrub to get rid of dead skin cells and product buildup.

- **Nutrition and Hydration:** Good hair begins on the inside. In order to support healthy hair growth, make sure you get plenty of water each day and eat a balanced diet full of vitamins and minerals like biotin, zinc, and vitamin E.

7.3 Dealing with Male Hair Loss

Men frequently experience hair loss, but it can be controlled with a variety of therapies, lifestyle changes, and acceptance of aging as a natural part of life. Knowing the options that are accessible to men who are experiencing baldness or hair thinning is essential for preserving their self-esteem and general well-being.

Male Pattern Baldness Treatment Options

A large percentage of males suffer from androgenetic alopecia, also known as male pattern baldness. Hair loss is mostly hereditary, but there are a few therapies that can halt or even reverse the process.

- **Minoxidil (Rogaine):** This over-the-counter topical medication increases blood flow to the scalp, which promotes the development of hair. In the initial phases of hair thinning, it works well.

- **Propecia, finasteride):** Finasteride is an oral prescription drug that functions by preventing testosterone from being converted into DHT, the hormone that causes male pattern baldness by causing hair follicles to shrink. Although it is a long-term remedy, results may not be seen for several months.

- **Hair Transplants:** Hair transplants provide a long-term remedy for males with more severe baldness. Hair follicles from the sides or back of the scalp are surgically transplanted to parts of the scalp that are losing hair.

- **Low-Level Laser Therapy (LLLT):** LLLT stimulates hair follicles with laser devices and has been proven to sometimes encourage regrowth.

Modifications to Lifestyle to Encourage Hair Growth

A few lifestyle adjustments can promote hair growth and enhance the general condition of existing hair. Including these adjustments in daily activities can stop additional hair loss and encourage regeneration.

1. **Well-Balanced Diet:** Make sure to consume a diet high in nutrients that promote healthy hair, like:
2. **Biotin:** This vitamin, which fortifies hair, is present in whole grains, eggs, and nuts.
3. **Omega-3 Fatty Acids:** Sourced from walnuts, flaxseed, and salmon, these fatty acids support healthy scalps.
4. **Protein:** Since keratin, a protein, is what makes hair, getting enough lean protein in your diet can help you grow hair.

Stress Management: Telogen effluvium, in particular, can cause hair loss due to elevated stress levels. Regular exercise, yoga, meditation, and other stress-reduction methods can help ward against this illness.

Avoiding Harsh Hair Treatments: Try to use as little chemicals such as relaxers and dyes as possible as these can weaken hair. Choose gentle methods and products to prevent harm to the hair and scalp.

Acknowledging Hair Loss

Accepting hair loss as a natural aspect of aging can be a powerful decision for many guys. A person's masculinity or attractiveness are not diminished by hair loss, and self-acceptance is the source of confidence.

- **Shaving the Head:** When hair loss becomes noticeable, many men find emancipation in shaving their entire head. Shaved heads are frequently viewed as daring and fashionable.

- **Grooming and Styling Short Hair:** Short, well-groomed haircuts can accentuate thinning hair and convey a polished impression for people who aren't ready for a shaved look.

- **Support and Confidence:** While some people may find hair loss emotionally taxing, it's crucial to concentrate on general health and confidence. Developing a positive self-image separate from one's hair can boost confidence.

Men's hair care include taking care of typical hair issues like hair loss as well as grooming and scalp health.

CHAPTER 8

Children's Hair Care

Children's hair demands careful attention to detail, taking into account the special textures and circumstances of growing hair. Children may be more susceptible to some hair problems and frequently have fragile scalps. This chapter delves into the fundamentals of hair care for kids, providing methods for mild cleaning, dealing with typical issues, and promoting good hair practices.

8.1 Taking Care of Kids' Hair

Children who receive proper hair care not only have healthier hair but also learn appropriate grooming skills at a young age. A caring attitude and gentle methods are essential to guaranteeing a satisfying hair care experience.

Mild Cleaning and Conditioning Methods

Since children's hair can be more fragile than adult hair, washing and conditioning it should be done with a gentler touch.

Selecting the Appropriate Products:
1. Make use of shampoos made especially for kids that are paraben and sulfate-free. These products minimize irritation by being kinder to the hair and scalp.
2. Select conditioners that are lightweight and simple to rinse off. Shampoos that contain natural components like chamomile or aloe vera help moisturize and calm the scalp.

Washing Frequency:
1. Washing 2-3 times a week is usually adequate for kids with fine hair. This keeps everything clean and helps avoid removing natural oils.
2. To avoid dryness and frizz, youngsters with thicker or curlier hair may only need to use this once a week.

Hand Washing Method:

1. Apply lukewarm water to cleanse hair, since hot water may cause skin sensitivity.

2. Instead of using your nails, gently massage the scalp from the roots to the ends using your fingertips.

3. Rinse well to get rid of all product residue, as it can cause irritation and accumulation.

Hair Detangling Advice for Kids

For both parents and children, detangling can be a difficult chore. This process can be streamlined and less stressful by employing the appropriate strategies.

- **Timing:** Work on detangling damp hair first because it's more manageable and malleable that way. To help loosen knots, use a detangling spray or leave-in conditioner.

Tools:

1. Use a kid-friendly detangling brush or a wide-toothed comb. These instruments lessen pain

and limit damage.

2. Work your way up to the roots by beginning to untangle from the ends. This technique makes it possible to work out knots softly and avoid pulling.

Patience: Teach kids to exercise patience when untangling. Assure them that it will become easier with practice by explaining the procedure.

Preventing Damage to Children's Hair

Improper care and environmental conditions can cause damage to children's hair. Taking preventative action can aid in keeping hair healthy.

Sun Protection:

1. Advise kids to cover up with hats or scarves when they spend a lot of time in the sun. UV rays can cause dryness and color fading in hair.

2. To offer even more protection, think about utilizing hair products with UV filters.

Heat Styling:

1. Keep children's hair away from heat styling appliances including curling irons, blow dryers, and straighteners. Use the lowest heat setting and a heat protectant if styling is required.

Dry Hair Caution:

1. Chlorine and seawater can cause dryness in hair. To reduce damage, rinse hair with fresh water both before and after swimming.
2. When using a pool, wear a swim cap to shield your hair from the chlorine.

8.2 Taking Care of Common Hair Problems in Kids

Numerous hair-related problems can arise in children, and taking quick action to address these issues can help to avoid more troubles and encourage healthy hair growth.

Frizzed Out and Dry Hair

Dry, frizzy hair is a common problem for kids, and it can be caused by dry air, dehydration, or poor hair care.

Moisturizing:

1. To enhance hydration and fight frizz, including deep conditioning treatments in their hair care regimen once a week. Look for products that contain coconut oil or shea butter, or other moisturizing components.

2. Apply a leave-in conditioner once a day to help keep moisture levels stable and lessen frizz.

Avoiding Excessive Washing: As was previously discussed, washing hair too regularly might remove its natural oils. Create a regimen that works for the type of hair on your child to keep it hydrated and nourished.

Natural Solutions: To counteract dryness and enhance manageability, a simple cure is to apply a tiny amount of natural oil (such as argan or jojoba oil) to the ends of the hair.

Prevention and Management of Head Lice

Children frequently worry about head lice, particularly in school environments. It is essential for parents to comprehend possibilities for prevention and treatment.

Preventive Measures:

1. Instruct kids not to share combs, hats, or other hair accessories because lice are spread by direct contact.

2. Promote routine hair inspections, particularly following playdates or sleepovers. Infestations can be avoided in large part by early identification.

Options for Treatment:

1. Use over-the-counter products made especially for treating head lice if any are found. For best results, please follow the directions.

2. To ensure that the scalp is lice-free, nits (lice eggs) must be removed by combining with a fine-toothed lice comb. Until all lice and nits are removed, this should be done every few days.

Children's Hair Loss

Although less often, medical disorders, stress, or inadequate diet can all contribute to hair loss in youngsters.

- **Determining the Root Cause:** Keep an eye out for any abrupt variations in hair thickness or areas where hair is missing. Alopecia areata, a disorder in which the immune system targets hair follicles, and telogen effluvium, a condition frequently brought on by stress or sickness, are examples of common causes.

Seeking Professional Help:

- See a dermatologist or pediatrician if hair loss is noticed. They can offer advice on suitable treatments and assist in identifying the underlying problem.

Social Assistance:

- For kids, hair loss can be upsetting. They can manage their emotions and keep a positive self-image with the assistance of emotional support and reassurance.

8.3 PROMOTING GOOD HAIR PRACTICES IN KIDS

The basis for lifetime hair care is laid by developing healthy hair habits early in childhood. Educating kids about hair care can help them develop a feeling of accountability and self-care.

Educating Kids on Hair Maintenance

Talks Regarding Education:

- Introduce the topic of hair care in an interesting and entertaining way. Explain the value of hygiene and upkeep using language and visuals that are appropriate for the audience's age.

- **Participation in Regular:** Invite kids to take part in their hair care regimen. Let children select the products for their own hair or offer assistance with cleaning and detangling. Being involved helps them become more independent and gives them a sense of pride in how their hair is cared for.

Positive Incentives and Reinforcement

- **Celebrating Progress:** Encourage kids to adopt good hair practices by providing them with positive reinforcement. Honor their accomplishments and efforts, no matter how modest.

Reward Systems:

- Create a system of rewards for regular hair care routines. Little rewards like stickers or more playtime can motivate kids to be proud of their personal hygiene routines.

Leadership by Example

- **As an example of behavior, consider:** The best way for kids to learn is through observation. You provide children a wonderful example to follow by taking good care of your hair yourself.

- **Hair Care Routine for the Family:** Think about starting a hair care regimen that the whole family can follow. This improves family ties while simultaneously reinforcing healthful behaviors.

More than simply basic grooming, taking care of children's hair also entails educating them, providing them with emotional support, and helping them form lasting habits.

Parents may help their children keep vibrant, healthy hair and inspire confidence that lasts a lifetime by using gentle ways, attending to common hair issues, and supporting healthy activities.

CHAPTER 9

Cost-Effective Hair Care

Keeping your hair healthy doesn't have to be expensive. You can stick to a budget and still create gorgeous, vivid hair with the correct strategies. This chapter covers a variety of cost-effective hair care techniques, such as making your own products and using smart buying strategies, so you have all the knowledge you need to maintain healthy hair without going over budget.

9.1 Homemade Hair Care Items

Making your own hair care products at home gives you control over the materials and can reduce costs. Customization is possible with DIY products, so you may meet your unique hair needs without having to pay extra for name brands.

Preparing DIY Hair Masks, Conditioner, and Shampoo

1. **Shampoo:** Castile soap, water, and essential oils are basic items that can be used to make an easy DIY shampoo. Hair can be effectively and gently cleaned with castile soap without losing its natural oils.

2. **Recipe:** To add scent and therapeutic advantages, mix one cup liquid castile soap, one cup water, and ten to fifteen drops of essential oil (such as lavender or tea tree).

Conditioner:

1. Natural ingredients like coconut oil, honey, and apple cider vinegar can be combined to quickly make a nutritious conditioner.

2. **Recipe:** Incorporate one tablespoon each of honey, apple cider vinegar, and coconut oil. Apply to damp hair, let it sit for ten to fifteen minutes, and then give it a good rinse.

Hair Masks:

1. Natural ingredient hair masks can help to deeply nourish and repair your hair. Yogurt, bananas, and

avocados are common ingredients that are high in vitamins and nutrients.

2. **Recipe:** One ripe banana should be mashed and combined with one tablespoon each of honey and olive oil. After applying the mixture to your hair, let it sit for 20 to 30 minutes before washing it out.

Using Natural Substances for Affordable Hair Care

Advantages of Using Natural Ingredients:

- Natural ingredients are less expensive and safer for your hair and scalp because they don't contain harsh chemicals. They are moisturizing and nourishing without posing a risk of irritation.

Some examples of effective ingredients are as follows:

1. **Olive Oil:** great for enhancing shine and hydrating.
2. **Honey:** An innate humectant that aids in moisture retention.
3. **Aloe Vera**: Encourages hair development and soothes the scalp.

Reducing Needless Expenses

- **Evaluation of Needs**: Consider your hair's demands and condition before making any purchases. By doing this, you'll avoid wasting money on products that might not be suitable for your hair type.

Multi-Functional Products:

- Seek out items that have more than one use, such leave-in conditioners that shield the sun or style lotions that nourish and retain hair.

9.2 Obtaining Reasonably Priced Hair Care Items

Finding high-quality hair care products at an affordable price can be accomplished through a variety of techniques. There are big savings to be had from wise purchasing.

Finding Discounts and Deals

When to Make Purchases: Shoppers should keep an eye out for seasonal discounts, clearance specials, and exclusive offers. Significant shopping occasions such as

Cyber Monday, Black Friday, and holiday sales frequently provide reduced prices on cosmetics and hair care items.

Bulk Buying:

- Take into account buying goods in large quantities. Long-term cost savings can be achieved by purchasing larger sizes or multipacks, which frequently lower the cost per unit.

Selecting Cost-Effective Brands

Looking for Alternatives:

- A lot of affordable brands provide high-quality goods that compete with more costly ones. Names like Herbal Essences, Garnier, and Suave offer high-quality hair care products at affordable prices.

Reading Reviews: Make use of internet resources to peruse evaluations and rankings concerning low-cost brands. By doing this, you may be confident that the products you're choosing are effective and avoid wasting money on useless ones.

Making Use of Discounts and Coupons

Where to Find Coupons:

- Look for coupons for hair care products on a regular basis via newspapers, websites, and shop circulars. Furthermore, a lot of firms provide coupons straight on their websites or in their newsletters.

- **Promotional Codes:** Look for coupons online that provide free shipping or discounts before making any purchases. These codes are compiled for convenience by websites such as Honey and RetailMeNot.

9.3 CUTTING HAIR TREATMENT COSTS

Professional hair treatments can be costly, but there are several ways to get salon-caliber results at home, which can cut down on the number of expensive salon trips.

Do-it-yourself hair coloring

- **Coloring Books for Home:** Take into consideration

employing simple and reasonably priced at-home hair coloring kits. Easy-to-use solutions from brands like Clairol and L'Oréal can yield excellent results for a fraction of the price of a salon visit.

- **Natural Hair Colors:** Look into natural hair coloring choices like vegetable dyes or henna. In the long term, these may be more cost-effective and are frequently safer for your hair and scalp.

Application Advice:

- Carefully read the directions and do a patch test prior to applying color to your full head. To get the greatest results, practice properly sectioning your hair for an even application.

At-Home Hair Curling and Straightening

- **Working with Styling Instruments:** Make an investment in long-lasting, high-quality styling equipment. You can avoid going to the salon by using a nice curling wand or straightening iron to produce the styles you want at home.

- **Styling Without Heat:** Think about styling your hair without the use of heat, like braiding wet hair for waves or spending the night with foam rollers. These techniques lessen heat damage and are reasonably priced.

Cutting Down on Salon Visits

- **Essential Trims at Home:** You can keep your hair looking nice in between professional trims by learning some fundamental haircutting techniques. With the correct equipment and a steady hand, simple trims can be completed at home.

Schedule Regular Maintenance:

- Arrange regular maintenance trims every 8–12 weeks in lieu of frequent salon visits. By doing this, you can maintain healthy hair without making as many salon visits.

Home Remedies:

- Include do-it-yourself remedies for typical problems

like frizz, dryness, and split ends. Frequent at-home maintenance helps preserve hair health and look while lowering the need for salon services.

You don't have to spend a fortune to have gorgeous, healthy hair if you follow these inexpensive tips. Whether you choose at-home treatments, thrifty shopping, or DIY hair care products, the important thing is to prioritize your hair's demands while keeping an eye on your budget. Even on a tight budget, you can get gorgeous hair with a little imagination and ingenuity.

CHAPTER 10

Special Occasion Hair Care

There are typically special occasion-specific requirements when it comes to hair maintenance and styling. Your whole appearance and confidence can be greatly enhanced by the way you prepare and take care of your hair, whether it's for a wedding, gala, or personal event. This chapter will cover the fundamentals of getting ready for events, taking care of your hair afterward, and special attention to important occasions such as weddings.

10.1 Hairstyling for Special Occasions

Preparing your hair for a particular occasion requires careful planning and style methods to make sure it looks flawless.

Healthy Hair Pre-Styling Treatments

- **Elucidating Interventions:** It's imperative to clarify your hair before style in order to get rid of product accumulation. To ensure a clean slate for styling, use a clarifying shampoo once a month to completely wash the scalp and hair.

- **Intense Conditioning:** One to two days prior to the event, give your hair a deep conditioning treatment to assist it maintain moisture and nourishment. To enhance the structure of your hair, choose protein-rich treatments like keratin masks.

- **Nutrition and Hydration:** To support healthy hair, eat a well-balanced diet high in vitamins and minerals. Foods rich in biotin, omega-3 fatty acids, and vitamins A, C, and E can support the health and radiance of hair.

Hairstyles and Updos for Various Occasions

Selecting the Appropriate Look: When choosing your haircut, take the event's formality into account. Elegant updos like braided buns or chignons are perfect for formal events. Loose waves or half-up styles could be more suitable for informal gatherings.

- **Experimental Runs:** Consider doing a trial run for a complicated hairstyle before committing to it. This lets you figure out what looks work best for you and guarantees that you have the appropriate tools and methods ready for the big day.

- **Including Current Trends:** Stay up to date with the latest hairstyle trends. Beachy waves, sleek ponytails, or curls with a retro vibe are other popular hairstyles. Modify these trends to suit the topic of the event and your own personal style.

Hairpieces and Styling Instruments

- **Choosing Accessory Items:** Your hairdo can be

greatly enhanced by adding hair accessories. Pick accessories like flower clips, combs, or colorful pins that will add flair and match your clothing. Make sure they are sturdy enough to endure the entire event.

Investing in Quality Tools:

- Make use of high-quality styling tools, like hair dryers with heat-adjustable settings, curling irons, and straighteners. Tools featuring ceramic or tourmaline technology can reduce heat damage while still producing good styling outcomes.

- List of Products Selected: Make an investment in hold-and-protect styling products including serums, hairspray, and mousse. To ensure a polished look without weighing down your hair, choose lightweight formulas.

10.2 HAIR CARE FOLLOWING SPECIAL OCCASIONS

It's essential to take good care of your hair after the excitement of a particular occasion in order to repair any potential damage from chemicals and styling.

Eliminating Styling Supplies and Remainder

- **Carefully Scrubbing:** To start, eliminate any product buildup from gels, sprays, and other styling products using a mild clarifying shampoo. This will assist in bringing back the luster and bounce of your hair.

Conditioning Procedures:

- To replenish moisture, use a deep conditioning mask or moisturizing conditioner afterward. To replenish your hair after an event, look for products that contain natural oils like argan or jojoba oil.

Nourishing and Deep Conditioning Your Hair

Daily Deep Conditioning:

- Include deep conditioning procedures in your regimen, particularly following noteworthy style occasions. This will keep the hair from becoming dry and brittle by repairing and hydrating it.

Leave-In Conditioners:

- Apply leave-in conditioners to maintain moisture levels and shield your skin from environmental aggressors. Between washing days, these can aid in preserving manageability and suppleness.

Keeping Your Hair Healthy Following Special Occasions

Careful Handling:

- Use caution when brushing or combing your hair after the event. Use a brush or wide-tooth comb that is meant to reduce breakage, particularly if your hair is wet.

- **Avoid Heat Styling:** Take a break from using heat styling equipment on your hair after the event. Accept styles that require no heat or air drying to help your hair heal.

- **Regular Trims:** To keep healthy growth and get rid of split ends, schedule regular trims. For your hair to stay vibrant and fresh-looking, aim for a haircut every 6 to 8 weeks.

10.3 WEDDING AND OTHER CELEBRATION HAIR CARE

Special attention to hair care is necessary for weddings and important celebrations to ensure that you look your best on these important occasions.

Wedding Hair Style Advice

Pre-Wedding Procedures:

- Start a special hair care routine three to six months before the wedding. For the best possible health for your hair, this entails routine haircuts, deep conditioning treatments, and eating a balanced diet.

- **Trial Hairstyles:** A few weeks before the wedding, set up a trial session for your bridal hairdo. This lets you try out different looks and tweak as necessary.

- **Introductory Professionals:** For the wedding day, think about bringing in a stylist with experience.

With their experience, you can look beautiful on your special day and worry less.

Hairdos for Particular Occasions

Think About the Theme:

- Select hairstyles that complement the celebration's theme. A modern wedding can require sleek, straight hairstyles or elaborate braids, but a vintage-themed wedding might look better with soft curls or a traditional updo.

- **Including Your Personal Style:** Make sure your hairdo conveys your sense of style and individuality. Your hair should be true to who you are, whether that means you like sophisticated, bohemian, or romantic styles.

Maintenance of Hair for Extended Hair Extensions

Selecting High-Quality Extensions: Select premium, ethically sourced hair that complements your natural texture and color if you decide to wear hair extensions.

This guarantees a realistic appearance and a smooth mix.

Maintenance Routine:

- Adhere to a certain maintenance regimen for your extensions, which can entail frequent conditioning, mild cleaning, and steering clear of extreme heat. To extend their life, think about utilizing specific products made for extensions.

- **Consulting Professionals:** To ensure that your extensions continue to look their best, seek application and upkeep advice from a qualified stylist. You can make sure your extensions stay in good shape by scheduling routine maintenance appointments.

Hair care for special occasions includes planning, maintenance after the event, and extra care for important events like weddings. By adhering to these recommendations, you can guarantee that your hair looks amazing and remains healthy, which will boost your self-esteem and allow you to fully enjoy these special times. By meticulously organizing and paying close attention to details, you can pull off a gorgeous appearance that amply elevates your special occasion.

ABOUT THE AUTHOR

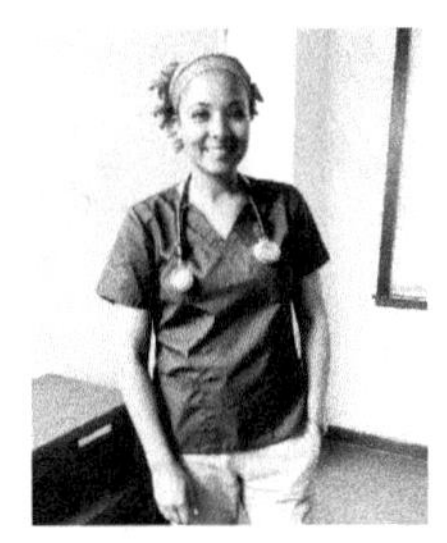

Harmony Royce is a dedicated healthcare worker who has a strong interest in holistic wellness. Harmony's extensive history in various aspects of health and wellness provides her with a wealth of knowledge and expertise that she can utilize in her writing and professional endeavors.

Harmony is a talented author who crafts thought-provoking books that inspire readers to have well-rounded, balanced lives. She writes about a variety of health-related topics, such as diet, exercise, mental health, and mindfulness. Her approachable writing style combines practical guidance with evidence-based research to make complex health concepts approachable and engaging for readers of all ages.

Harmony actively promotes the benefits of holistic health through writing, community workshops, and internet forums. Her mission is to educate and inspire people about the transformative power of self-care and healthy lifestyle choices.